FAQ

TEEN LIFE™

FREQUENTLY ASKED QUESTIONS ABOUT

Cancer Decisions for You and Your Family

Colleen
Ryckert
Cook

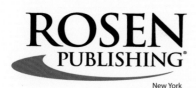

ROSEN
PUBLISHING®

New York

616.994
COO

Published in 2011 by The Rosen Publishing Group, Inc.
29 East 21st Street, New York, NY 10010

Library of Congress Cataloging-in-Publication Data

Cook, Colleen Ryckert.
Frequently asked questions about cancer decisions for you and your family / Colleen Ryckert Cook.—1st ed.
    p. cm.—(FAQ: teen life)
Includes bibliographical references and index.
ISBN 978-1-4488-1326-1 (libr. bdg.)
1. Cancer—Popular works. I. Title.
RC263.C6486 2011
616.99'4—dc22

                                                          2010018501

Manufactured in the United States of America

CPSIA Compliance Information: Batch #W11YA: For further information, contact Rosen Publishing, New York, New York, at 1-800-237-9932.

Contents

one

I HAVE CANCER. WHAT HAPPENS NOW?

In the next months, you and your family will focus on learning all you can about your cancer. Your existence will seem to revolve around oncologist appointments. You'll get so used to having blood drawn that you won't even flinch at needles. In no time, you'll rattle off four- and five-syllable medical terms like a pro. You'll probably memorize the names of entire nursing staffs.

It's difficult, scary, and lonely. You probably feel like you're the only teen in the world dealing with cancer. The truth is lots of other teens and even younger children are going through the same thing. The National Cancer Institute's Surveillance and Epidemiology and End Results (SEER) program gathers cancer statistics in America. According to SEER's most recent estimates, more than forty-seven thousand children and teens live with cancer each year. Many have dealt with it for five years or more. This year alone, about eighteen thousand will hear the words "you have cancer" for the first time.

Remember how you felt when you heard you had cancer? You're probably still processing what this means. It takes time. Some teens are scared at first. Others are convinced the doctors were wrong. Some want to hide or don't want friends to know. And some feel determined to beat cancer fast.

Nearly every single teen with cancer will tell you the same thing. During long months and even years of treatment, they ride a roller coaster of emotions. Depending on the day and sometimes even the hour, they feel frustrated, joyful, dismal, goofy, angry, hopeful, and often, believe it or not, bored.

Why Did I Get Cancer?

The simple response: the deoxyribonucleic acid, or DNA, changed in some of your cells, which allowed them to grow out of control. Those cells no longer function properly.

Our bodies have tumor-suppressor genes. These genes slow down cell division and help repair DNA errors. They also tell cells to die off to make room for new cells. Different genes, called proto-oncogenes, control cell function and division. Mutated proto-oncogenes are called oncogenes. Oncology, or the study of cancer, comes from this word. If oncogenes grow out of control or tumor-suppressor genes stop working, the result is cancer.

We know prolonged exposure to certain things can cause cancer. We call them carcinogens. Common carcinogens include

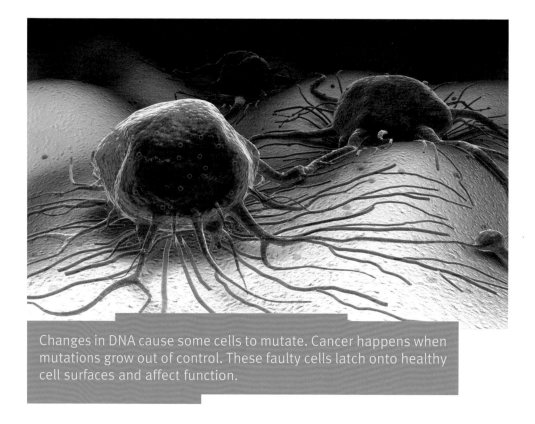

Changes in DNA cause some cells to mutate. Cancer happens when mutations grow out of control. These faulty cells latch onto healthy cell surfaces and affect function.

asbestos, cigarettes and second-hand smoke, coal tar, hepatitis C, polychlorinated biphenyls (PCBs), radon, and ultraviolet rays and X-rays.

Your cells might have a predisposition, passed down in your family, to mutate. Many mutations develop in embryos or show up shortly after birth. Some pop up decades later to catch every-one by surprise.

For whatever reason, something went wrong inside your cells. Remember those cellular mitosis lessons from science class? Each time a mutated cell divides to create a new cell, the mutation repeats. Over time, a mass of altered cells forms.

Sometimes these masses, or tumors, are benign. They're in the way but harmless. Other tumors, like what you're dealing with, are malignant. They make an impact on the cells around them. The body can't function the way it should.

What Kinds of Cancers Do Teens and Children Develop?

"Cancer" is a blanket term for hundreds of diseases. Leukemia, or cancer of the white blood cells, is the most common malignancy that affects children. According to the National Cancer Institute, leukemia accounts for about thirty-three out of every one hundred childhood cancer diagnoses. Brain tumors, non-Hodgkin's lymphoma, soft tissue cancers, and Hodgkin's lymphoma are the other most frequently occurring cancers in people under age twenty.

For young people between the ages of seven and sixteen, however, bone and soft tissue cancers (called sarcomas) are more common. This is because the body goes through growth spurts during those years: bone and soft tissue cells multiply quickly during puberty as an adolescent's body matures.

Your doctors will provide information for your specific cancer, but here is some general information from the National Cancer Institute and SEER about common cancers in older children and teens.

Leukemia

Leukemia is a blood cancer that causes bone and joint pain, bleeding, weight loss, fatigue, and other symptoms. The most common type is acute lymphoblastic leukemia (ALL), which accounts for about 80 percent of childhood leukemias. Acute myelogenous leukemia (AML) accounts for about 20 percent of childhood leukemias, although a few other rare forms also exist. Although childhood leukemia sounds really scary, the overall five-year survival rates are actually now between 80 percent and 85 percent. This means children diagnosed with leukemia were treated successfully (in remission) and are alive five years later.

Brain Tumors

Brain tumors are the next most common cancer of childhood. These tumors can appear anywhere in the brain or spine, but most often occur in the brain stem (where the spinal cord joins the back of the brain) or cerebellum (an area of the back of the brain that coordinates movement). Symptoms depend on where the tumor pops up. They can include trouble with speaking, vomiting, headaches, vision problems, seizures, coordination problems, numbness, weakness, and personality changes.

There are many different types of brain tumors, and they are named for the type of cell from which they arose and sometimes by their location. About half of all childhood brain tumors are called astrocytomas, which can be low grade (benign) or high grade (malignant). These tumors develop from astrocytes, which are supporting cells (glia) within the brain and spinal cord. These tumors tend to look spindly and can spread easily into healthy tissue. This can make them hard to remove surgically. Other common brain tumors are called primitive neuroectodermal tumors (PNETs) because they start in primitive (immature) nerve cells. PNETs account for about 20 percent of childhood brain tumors. Medulloblastoma is a kind of PNET. There are also dozens of other less common central nervous system tumors.

Many brain tumors in children are called indolent, which means the tumors grow slowly. Other tumors grow more quickly, such as anaplastic astrocytomas and glioblastomas multiforme (the most aggressive type of astrocytoma). Depending on the type and location, brain tumors are treated with surgery, radiation, and/or chemotherapy.

Lymphomas

Lymphomas account for about 10 percent of all childhood cancers. They can develop almost anywhere because the lymphatic system runs throughout the body. Common sites include the neck, chest, armpits, spleen, thymus, adenoid and tonsils, intestines, and bone marrow. Boys tend to develop lymphomas more than girls. These diseases are usually detected as swollen lymph nodes in the neck, armpit, or groin. Lymphomas can cause fever, sweating, itchiness, weakness, and weight loss in some people. This type of cancer is usually treated with chemotherapy and radiation.

Non-Hodgkin's lymphoma (NHL) and Hodgkin's lymphoma, also called Hodgkin's disease (HD), occur at about the same rates. Non-Hodgkin's lymphoma usually occurs in younger children, though, while HD is more likely to affect older children and adolescents.

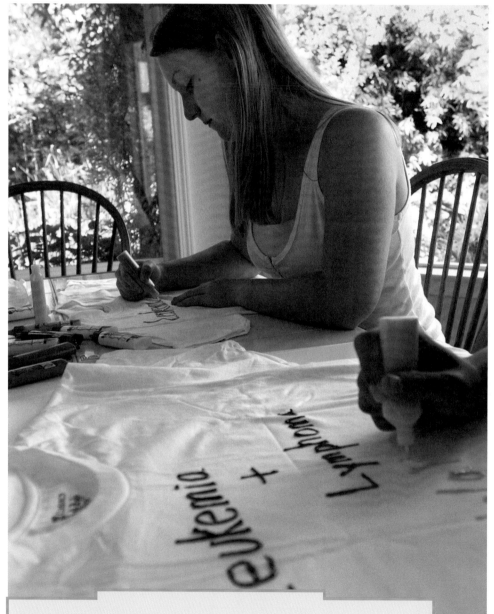

Teens decorate shirts for a cancer research walk-a-thon. About 43 percent of children diagnosed with cancer will have some form of leukemia or lymphoma.

Lymphoblastic lymphomas (a type of NHL) account for 30 percent of all childhood lymphomas and are most common in teenagers. They grow and can spread to other parts of the body, often to the bone marrow and lymph nodes in the chest. Boys develop this kind of cancer twice as often as girls do. Large cell lymphomas, which are much less common, tend to grow more slowly and aren't as likely to spread to other parts of the body. There are several other less common forms of NHL.

HD rarely develops in children younger than five years old, but is most common in teens and young adults (as well as older people in their fifties and sixties). Young adults with HD most commonly develop the nodular sclerosis form, which shows up in the neck or chest. There are other types of HD that are less common in children and teens.

Bone Cancer

When you hear about someone with bone cancer, it does not necessarily mean that the cancer first showed up in the person's bone cells. It may have started in other cells of the body and metastasized, or spread, to the bones. Cancer that actually starts in the bones is called primary bone cancer and is quite uncommon. Not long ago, bone tumors meant amputation. In many cases nowadays, doctors can save healthy bone around a tumor. Metal rods and pins act as bones or joints.

Children tend to develop two forms of primary bone cancer. Osteosarcomas are the most common form and account for about 3 percent of all childhood cancers in the United States.

This type of tumor most commonly develops in the long bones near the knees. The upper arm near the shoulder is the next most common site, but these tumors can form in hips, elbows, jaws—anywhere bones grow. Osteosarcoma is usually treated with intensive chemotherapy and surgery.

Ewing's sarcoma, the next most common bone cancer in children and teens, accounts for slightly more than 1 percent of all childhood cancers. It mostly happens in children between ten and twenty years old. This sarcoma responds well to radiation and is also treated with chemotherapy and surgery.

Sarcomas

Cancers of connective tissues, such as muscle or fat, are called sarcomas. These tumors can happen anywhere in the body. The most common soft tissue sarcoma in children is called rhabdomyosarcoma (RMS). It accounts for about 350 new cases each year and comes in a few types. Embryonal RMS is the most common (about 75 percent) and mostly happens in younger children, while alveolar RMS is less common and affects children and teens equally. Embryonal RMS tends to occur in the head and neck areas. Alveolar RMS occurs most often in the arms and legs, then the head and neck. RMS is usually treated with chemotherapy, surgery, and/or radiation.

Where Can I Get Help?

There are cancer centers around the country that specialize in childhood cancer. Professionals at these centers know how

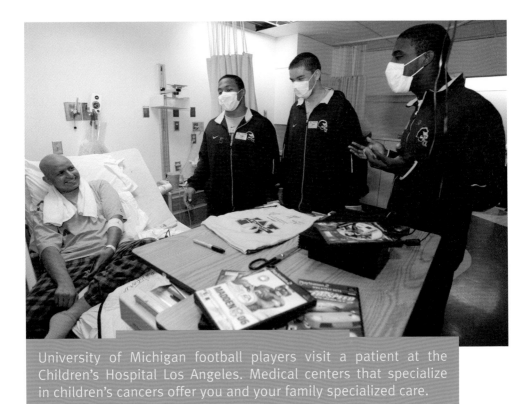

University of Michigan football players visit a patient at the Children's Hospital Los Angeles. Medical centers that specialize in children's cancers offer you and your family specialized care.

cancer differs in children and the best method for treating these patients. Childhood cancers are usually very different from adult cancers and so need different treatments.

You'll hear the phrase "five-year survival rates" a lot when doctors talk about treatment options. The goal is to eliminate cancer cells and keep you in remission, or cancer-free, for years to come. Doctors treat childhood cancers with a combination of surgery, radiation, and chemotherapy, depending on the type of cancer. Some patients may also need immunotherapy to boost damaged immune systems. Your treatment plan depends on your cancer: its type, stage, location, and even the unique way your cells respond to it.

Cancer treatments damage the body's fastest-growing cells the most. These include mouth and throat tissues, hair follicles, and the stomach and intestines. That's why people develop mouth sores, lose their hair, or feel sick to their stomachs.

The good news: Most childhood cancers respond to chemotherapy and radiation, and young people generally tolerate the side effects much better than adults do. There are risks with any treatment, of course, which should be thoroughly explained to you. Doctors will provide paperwork called informed consent forms. This paperwork explains your condition, what your specific treatment plan will do for your cancer, any side effects or risks, and other treatment options.

If you are eligible for participation in a clinical trial, your doctor will explain this treatment option as well. Participating in a clinical trial does not mean that the doctors are experimenting on you or that you'll be a guinea pig. It simply means that you could receive a new therapy or a new way to administer cancer treatments that might improve the cure rate even more. Because childhood cancer is rare, hospitals across the country put their resources together to figure out the best way to treat children and teens with various cancers. As a result of these clinical trials, cure rates for many childhood cancers have gotten much better over the years.

You and your parents should read everything your doctors provide and get answers to all of your questions before you sign the paperwork. Look at the probable outcome versus potential complications. The more you understand, the more informed your decision will be.

Childhood cancer facilities also offer psychological and nutritional services for families. You can meet with social workers, child life specialists, and rehabilitation and physical therapists. There are even teachers who will help you keep up with schoolwork. They know how to treat the emotional and physical needs that sick teens and children have. You and your family have important decisions to make, and these trained and experienced people can help.

Families who've dealt with childhood cancer can help you during the first difficult months. Talk to them. Your cancer center can suggest local groups or even pair you up with another family from your cancer center.

two

WHAT SHOULD WE KNOW ABOUT SURGICAL TREATMENT?

Surgery is the first choice if doctors believe they can safely remove a tumor, although patients may also need chemotherapy and/or radiation. In a few cases, surgeons can excise the mass and that's it—no follow-up chemo or radiation.

Most patients with solid cancers require more than one kind of treatment. Chemotherapy can be used prior to surgery to shrink a tumor so that the surgery can be performed more easily. Chemotherapy and/or radiation can also be used after surgery to kill any remaining cancer cells in the area of the tumor itself, as well as any cells that may have escaped (metastasized). Leukemia and lymphoma patients don't need surgery to treat their cancers, although many patients with cancer go through a brief surgery to put in a special kind of IV called a

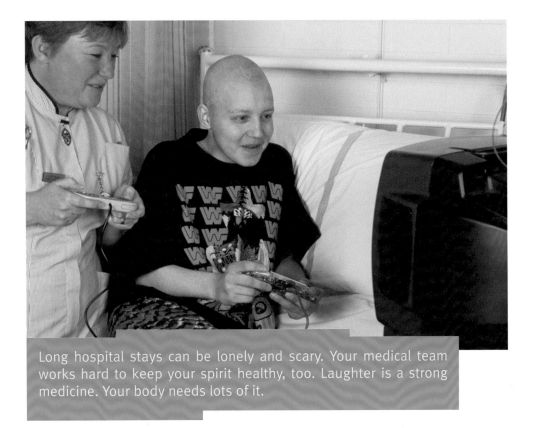

Long hospital stays can be lonely and scary. Your medical team works hard to keep your spirit healthy, too. Laughter is a strong medicine. Your body needs lots of it.

central venous catheter. These central venous catheters make it easier for doctors to give you chemotherapy or draw blood. It's better for you in the long run because you don't have to be stuck with a needle every time you need treatment or tests. It is also safer to give most chemotherapy through catheters into the bigger veins of your chest, rather than the tiny ones in your hands or arms.

Many lymphomas and solid tumors must be diagnosed by biopsy, which is a type of minor surgery in which a sample of the suspect tissue is removed with a thin needle. This tissue is then examined by a pathologist, a doctor who studies tissues to help make diagnoses. A biopsy tells your oncologist exactly what kind of cancer you have and what it looks like under the microscope. This information can help doctors stage your cancer in some cases.

Staging is a ranking system that oncologists use to create the best treatment plan for your cancer. Each cancer type is staged differently and specifically by its particular characteristics. With solid tumors, stage depends mostly upon size and whether the cancer has spread. Doctors also grade the aggressiveness of tumor cells by how they look under the microscope. Grade 1 means the tumor is the least aggressive type. Grade 4 is the most aggressive. With leukemia and lymphoma, doctors look at other factors like genetic changes within the cancer cells to determine proper treatment plans. Your doctor will explain the details of your cancer stage and grade.

Before Surgery

Some people get diagnosed one day and are in the hospital the following morning. Families have little time to think about the decisions they must make. It also isn't unusual to wait a few weeks before surgery. This can seem even more stressful, but extra time is a good thing. You can prepare your body with nutrient-rich food and exercise if your doctor says it's OK. You can prepare your mind by learning about your cancer. Your parents can take care of insurance and preapprovals. And you can get answers to all of your questions.

Surgery risks include reactions to anesthesia, bleeding and possible transfusions, or damage to organs or surrounding tissue. Remember those tests you took to get your diagnosis? You'll need more before surgery. Blood tests check cell counts, your blood's ability to clot, and the function of organs like the kidney and liver. Urinalysis also checks kidney function. X-rays or other studies such as ultrasound, CT scans, PET scans, or MRIs look at your tumor and any possible sites of spread. You may have other tests, depending on your type of cancer. Ask your doctor about what will happen during a test and why you need it.

You will meet most, if not all, of the team that will be with you during your operation. You'll meet your pediatric surgeon, anesthesiologist, and nurses. Depending on your surgery, you might also have an orthopedic surgeon, neurosurgeon, plastic surgeon, or even a dental surgeon.

At the Hospital

Some small procedures, such as certain biopsies, require only a topical anesthesia. It is similar to what you get at the dentist. Doctors numb a small part of your body, either with an injection or cream. They use a tiny needle to penetrate the tumor and withdraw some cells. You can be done in an hour or so.

When it comes to cancer, most surgical procedures require stronger stuff. Regional anesthesia is a nerve block, which completely numbs the area of interest for the biopsy, but allows you to stay awake. The person who gives you this medicine is an anesthesiologist. He or she may numb just your arm or leg, or

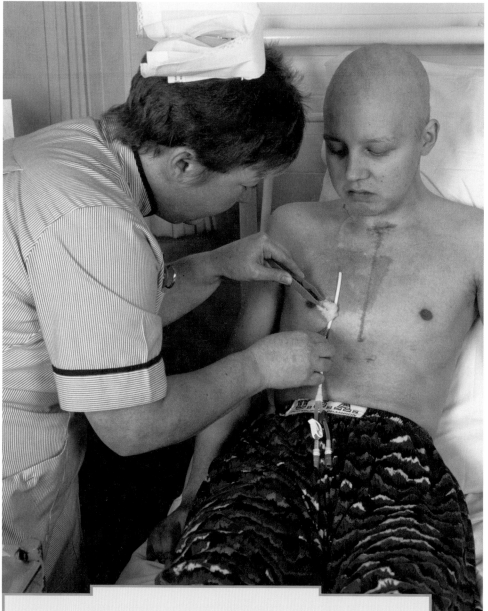

Central venous catheters make getting treatments or blood tests much easier on cancer patients. Catheters are surgically inserted under the skin and must be kept clean.

you may need a nerve block that is given in the spine and will numb everything from your waist down.

Most actual cancer surgeries to remove tumors require general anesthesia, though. Special drugs put you into a deep sleep. Doctors will insert an endotracheal tube into your throat to help you breathe. You can't eat for several hours before general anesthesia. That's because there is a small chance you might vomit while you're in surgery. This can be dangerous because you can't cough it out. Fasting before surgery lessens this chance. Your anesthesiologist will monitor your heart, breathing, and blood pressure the entire time. Nurses and your surgeon will look out for you, too.

Sometimes doctors leave a tiny tube that juts out from the incision site. This is called a drain, and it drains fluid to help you heal faster. You might need a drain for a few days or longer. Once it stops collecting fluid, your doctor will remove it.

When you wake up after surgery, you'll feel woozy for a while. Some people throw up. After regional or general anesthesia, doctors will observe you for several hours or overnight to make sure the effects of the anesthesia wear off properly. The goal is to get you moving and on solid foods as soon as safely possible.

You might not want to get out of bed at first, but it's important for several reasons. It gets your blood moving, which lowers the risk of developing clots in your blood vessels. Exercise makes your lungs work normally, and this reduces your chances of developing a lung infection such as pneumonia. Doctors will give you medicine to help ease pain so that you can get moving.

Surgery puts you at risk for developing a lung infection, such as pneumonia. After surgery, some patients use tools like this volumetric exerciser to make sure their lungs are working hard.

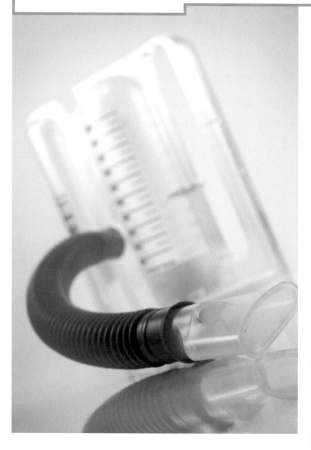

Moving also helps your digestive system return to normal. General anesthesia makes it sluggish. If you can't digest food properly, you might develop a blockage in your intestines. In the worst case, you might need more surgery to get rid of the blockage. You need a healthy digestive system to absorb nutrients. It might seem embarrassing to pass gas in public, but it's a goal after surgery. Often, you can't leave the hospital until you have a bowel movement.

If you can't get out of bed, doctors will have you do deep breathing exercises. One tool is a plastic tube with a small ball inside. You blow as hard as you can into a mouthpiece to force the ball to rise. A rehabilitation therapist will exercise your limbs.

Back Home

When it's time to leave the hospital, you'll receive instructions about pain management, diet restrictions, and rehabilitation exercises. Infection is a risk, so the nurses will teach you how to care for your incision and any drain or catheter. Ask lots of questions and make sure you understand everything before you go home.

How fast you recover depends on many things. You might feel back to your usual self in a few days. It might take longer. People who have brain or bone surgeries may need months of physical rehabilitation to relearn tasks or use a prosthetic limb. Some patients might have a catheter, feeding tube, or colostomy bag. Adjusting to dramatic body changes takes time.

It's also likely that you'll be facing several weeks, months, or even years of additional treatment. You might need future surgeries. This can be a scary, uncertain time. Your doctors, nurses, child life specialists, rehabilitation therapists, and social workers can help you and your family.

three

WHAT SHOULD I KNOW ABOUT RADIATION TREATMENTS?

The same high-level rays that can cause cells to turn cancerous can also kill them effectively. Radiation is often used to treat brain and spinal cord tumors, rhabdomyosarcomas, Ewing's sarcomas, and some lymphomas.

Radiation continues to kill cancerous cells for weeks, even months, after the last treatment. It works because healthy cells recover more quickly than cancer cells do. The damaged cells can't handle the assault and die off before they can spread. In best-case scenarios, tumors shrink and disappear.

Radiation can be used to target tumors precisely and minimize damage to healthy cells. Sometimes doctors use radiation to treat sites where the tumors are completely gone, but have a high risk of returning. Radiation

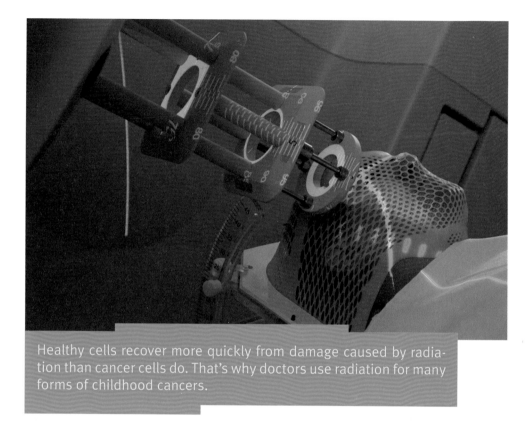

Healthy cells recover more quickly from damage caused by radiation than cancer cells do. That's why doctors use radiation for many forms of childhood cancers.

treatment can also relieve pain from tumors pushing on nerves in the body.

What Are the Different Kinds of Radiation?

Doctors can deliver radiation treatments externally or internally. Most patients receive low-dose treatments several days a week for a certain length of time. This might last weeks or longer. Many cancers respond to lower doses over a longer time period, but some need intensive treatment with larger doses over a shorter period of time. Your doctor will choose the best plan for your cancer.

Conformal radiation therapy is a highly focused external beam treatment given in daily increments. It can be high-dose or low-dose radiation. This helps spare surrounding healthy tissue as much as possible.

Radiosurgery (also known as gamma knife) is a single high-dose external treatment directed to a small region of the brain. The dose is five to ten times larger than a typical daily dose. Doctors attach a neurosurgical frame to the patient's head. This keeps the head still to focus the radiation precisely on the tumor and spare healthy tissue.

Brachytherapy is a form of internal radiation. Radioactive isotopes are sealed into a holder called an implant, which is placed in the body through a surgical procedure. Implants might be thin wires, catheters, capsules, or seeds. They can be temporary or permanent.

Total body irradiation (TBI) is a body-wide internal treatment and is often given in combination with chemotherapy. TBI prepares diseased bone marrow for the transplant of healthy blood-forming cells. Patients must stay in the hospital for several weeks to months to prepare for and recover from bone marrow transplantation.

What Happens During Treatment?

With brachytherapy, surgeons place a catheter implant under the skin at or near the tumor site. About five to six days later, the

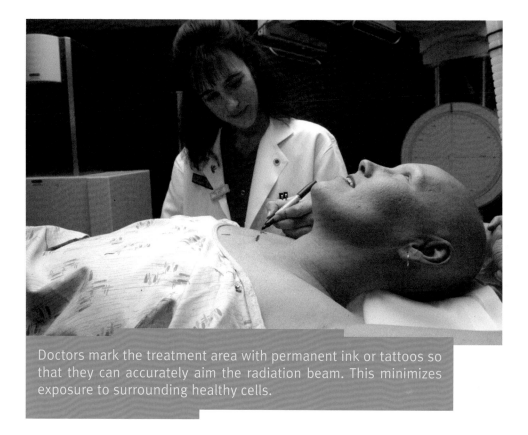

Doctors mark the treatment area with permanent ink or tattoos so that they can accurately aim the radiation beam. This minimizes exposure to surrounding healthy cells.

radiologist fills the implant with isotopes. Most implants are temporary. Doctors will remove an implant after the radiation course ends. This can last several days. In some cases, implants are permanent. They remain harmless in the body after radiation ends and eventually dissolve away.

External beam radiation treatments are done at a radiology clinic. Radiologists use equipment similar to an X-ray machine. Your first appointment will be a dress rehearsal. The radiologist will take MRIs or X-rays to pinpoint tumors, then use permanent ink to mark or perhaps tattoo the target site.

After you're settled comfortably in the treatment chair, the radiologist will adjust the machine to the proper angle. Exact measurements make sure the radiation team can set up the equipment correctly for future appointments. This first visit can last up to two hours. Your first treatment can take up to one hour, but the rest usually last only ten to fifteen minutes. Getting radiation itself does not hurt, although it can cause some unpleasant side effects.

Your cancer team will monitor you throughout treatment. Sometimes solid tumors look bigger on X-rays after you start radiation. That's because the rays can inflame cells and cause swelling. This will shrink in time.

Radiation also weakens your immune system. As a result, you may be more susceptible to infections. However, antibiotics will help you fight them. Your treatment team will want you to call if you develop a fever. Sometimes doctors will hospitalize radiation patients until their white blood counts hit the healthy range.

What Are the Side Effects and Risks?

Better technology means cancer patients get more focused radiation therapy than was possible in the past. There are still risks, though. Factors that have nothing to do with radiation can make a difference as to how you feel, too. Poor nutrition makes it harder for your body to recover from treatment. You might feel worse if surgery damaged surrounding tissue. And some people just react badly to radiation.

Short-term side effects show up within days or weeks of treatment. Common complaints include skin discoloration or a burn similar to sunburn. Some patients feel weak. Problems can pop up near the treatment site. For example, radiation for a hip tumor might cause diarrhea because the radiation can affect the intestines. Brain cancer patients might lose their hair. Side effects are generally localized to the treatment site. Most side effects go away after treatment ends.

What Are Late Effects?

Late effects are complications that can show up months or even years after treatment stops. Your risks depend on lots of factors: your age, your cancer, how healthy you were before cancer, and other factors.

Like radiation's short-term effects, late effects often show up at or near the treatment site. These include permanent damage called tissue atrophy, scarring, pigmentation damage, and secondary cancers. Children who received radiation for brain tumors may have learning problems and damage to the endocrine system. This can cause poor growth, urinary issues, and thyroid issues.

Radiation to the torso can lower your lung capacity or damage your heart. Some brain or eye cancer patients might suffer hearing loss or vision problems, such as cataracts or night blindness. Radiation near the face can alter facial shape in growing children. It can also cause dental problems, such as damaged enamel or tooth decay.

For children and teens, muscle and bone cells are especially vulnerable to cancer treatments. Late effects from radiation can include osteoporosis (weak bones), stiff joints, inflamed cartilage, uneven growth, or gait problems.

Radiation of the brain or other organs can also damage the endocrine system. This includes the pituitary, thyroid, and adrenal glands and depends on the site of radiation. Patients might experience stunted growth or learning disabilities. In many cases, doctors can shield you to minimize damage. Talk to your doctor about risks and how to best protect healthy cells.

Myths and Facts

Cell phones, hair dyes, deodorants, and diet sodas cause cancer. Fact ➡ In extremely large quantities, certain chemicals can cause cancer. Such exposure does not happen on a daily basis, however. Radiation can increase cancer risks for the same reasons. It's highly unlikely that people get cancer because they text all the time, dye their hair, or drink four diet sodas a day.

Exposure to high-frequency ionizing radiation—such as gamma rays and X-rays—can change cellular DNA, which can lead to cancer. Cell phones and microwaves emit low-frequency radiation. The American Cancer Society states that those fields are unlikely to cause DNA changes.

Studies in the 1970s found chemicals in hair dyes caused cancers in animals. Manufacturers changed the ingredients. The National Cancer Institute says there is no clear evidence linking modern dye formulations to cancer.

The National Cancer Institute also says there isn't conclusive evidence linking aluminum compounds in deodorants and antiperspirants to breast cancers. It found no definitive links between sweeteners and cancers in humans, either. Still, you could find healthier choices than diet sodas to quench your thirst.

 Cancer is contagious. Fact ⇒ This myth probably hangs around because certain viruses can lead to cancer. Some types of human papillomavirus (HPV) cause cervical cancers. Hepatitis C can cause liver cancers. Theses viruses are contagious, but not everyone who gets the viruses develops cancers.

There are genetic links to certain types of cancer, but you didn't catch it from anyone in your family, either. Some cells in your body changed, for whatever reason, but they won't cause the cells of those you love to change.

 Biopsies can cause cancer to spread. Fact ⇒ In the past, doctors used larger needles for biopsies. There was a risk of leaking cancerous cells into the bloodstream to further mutate. Nowadays, oncologists use fine needles to reduce damage and minimize risks. Still, some doctors won't biopsy certain cancers, such as testicular or eye cancer. They may opt to treat the tumor as if it's malignant or instead remove it entirely. Talk to your doctor about any concerns.

four

WHAT HAPPENS IF I NEED CHEMOTHERAPY?

Often when people hear they need chemotherapy, they become afraid. Chemotherapy works for most patients, though, and many children remain cancer-free for the rest of their lives.

Chemotherapy is a systemic, or body-wide, treatment. Your doctors might call it antineoplastic (anticancer) or cytotoxic (cell-killing) therapy. There are more than one hundred different kinds of cancer drugs available. It's rare for doctors to use only one medicine. More likely, your oncologist will prescribe a combination of different medicines to treat your unique cancer. They often call this mix a cocktail.

You'll also likely take other medications throughout treatment to prevent infections, help with nausea and vomiting, and support your immune system.

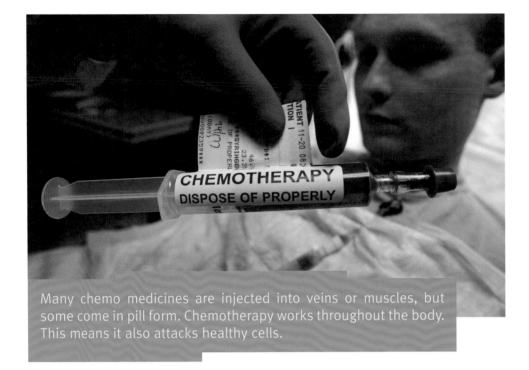

Many chemo medicines are injected into veins or muscles, but some come in pill form. Chemotherapy works throughout the body. This means it also attacks healthy cells.

Using a combination of chemotherapy agents attacks cancer cells from multiple angles and can prevent them from developing drug resistance. Combination chemotherapy also reduces the chance of toxicity buildup. Everyone metabolizes drugs differently, so your doctors will monitor you closely. They want to find the most effective combination without wreaking too much havoc on your healthy cells.

What Happens During Treatment?

Many chemo drugs are given intravenously because this is the most effective method for targeting and killing cancer cells. There are certain drugs that doctors must inject directly into a muscle or even the tumor site. Some chemo drugs come in pill form.

Like radiation, chemo damages your immune system. Antibiotics help fight infections. Even with IV chemo, it isn't unusual to take a dozen pills several times a day. You should always talk with your doctor about any other medicines, vitamins, or supplements that you might want to take. Some of these can be dangerous or interfere with your chemotherapy.

For IV treatments, doctors often use central venous catheters. These are surgically inserted under general anesthesia, usually into a large vein in the torso. The catheters or ports stay in place until the final treatment. This can last for months or even years.

There are two main types of central venous catheters. One type, often called a Broviac or Hickman catheter, hangs outside the body. It's strange at first, having a tube dangle off your chest, but it will make getting treatment much easier. Doctors simply hook you up to a pump that delivers the medicine. You don't need an IV line inserted each time.

A second type, called a Port-a-Cath, is inserted under the skin. This gives you the freedom to do more activities, like swim. They aren't the best option for some cancer types. Also, you must endure a needle prick to access the port for treatment. Your doctor will recommend the best type of catheter for your cancer and your treatment plan.

It's especially important during any cancer treatment to take your medicines on schedule, even if it means waking up in the middle of the night to take a pill. You might take some meds on an empty stomach and others with food. Things can get complicated when you're taking several pill combinations throughout the day. A schedule posted on your refrigerator or cabinet door can remind you what you need to do.

Because of possible interactions, you'll get a list of things you can and can't take by mouth. These can include over-the-counter medications like aspirin and ibuprofen. Never take any drug, even those you can buy at a grocery store, during chemo treatment unless your doctor approves it. Keep an updated list of all medications, including your chemo combinations. Things can change fast. It's important that you update the list each time your drugs or dosages change. Your doctors will want to see the list at every appointment.

Doctors will examine you often during treatment. They will test your blood and check any tumors for changes. Chemo can be hard on the body. Some medicines are worse than others. You can help yourself by eating nutrient-rich foods, getting lots of rest, and trying to exercise a little. The healthier your body is, the better you'll be able to fight off chemo's damage.

Your oncologist does more than just take care of your cancer. You'll have to answer lots of questions about how you're feeling about everything, from parents to algebra to your friends. A whole team of doctors and nurses want to help your family as you manage this upheaval. Attitude matters when it comes to how your body feels. You'll have bad days. A sense of humor and a positive outlook can get you through those rough times.

Chemo's Side Effects

Chemotherapy unfortunately may interfere with the development and function of healthy cells. This causes the side effects

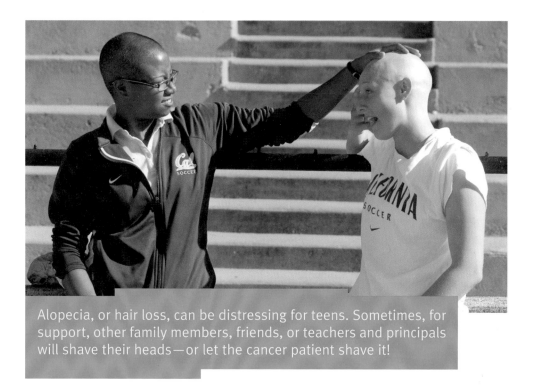

Alopecia, or hair loss, can be distressing for teens. Sometimes, for support, other family members, friends, or teachers and principals will shave their heads—or let the cancer patient shave it!

you often hear about. How you respond can depend on the combination and quantities of drugs used, how healthy you were before you started chemo, your attitude, even life at school or home.

Specific side effects depend on what type of chemotherapy you are getting. Some chemotherapies cause mouth sores. Your gums might look pale or bleed. Food can taste different. For example, lots of people say chemo causes sweet foods to taste metallic. Chemo can wipe out red blood cells, which leads to anemia. Anemic people tire quickly, can be short of breath, and can have high heart rates.

Lots of people feel nauseated and lose their appetites. Some develop constipation, diarrhea, or both. Some people find they're hungry all the time. Some people lose weight because they feel sick or food doesn't taste good. Others gain weight, have trouble sleeping, and may have behavior problems while taking steroid chemotherapies.

Some people have allergic reactions or break out in rashes. Some develop alopecia, which means they lose all their hair. Others only deal with thinning hair. A few don't notice a difference.

Certain chemo drugs can harm heart cells. Some people develop swollen hands or feet because they are retaining water. This is called edema. Some people might feel dizzy or have an erratic heartbeat. Some children experience slowed growth.

Hormone imbalances can cause irregular or missed periods. Treatment can delay or speed up the start of puberty or cause early menopause in adulthood. Sometimes puberty stops before a child is fully developed.

Medicines can help with most stomach troubles. Lotions soothe irritated skin. Moist swabs, hard candies, or rinses relieve inflamed mouth tissues. Hats, scarves, or wigs make some people more comfortable about hair loss.

Side effects usually end once the chemicals leave your body, but some are permanent. Growth rates usually return to normal, but you might not catch up to where you could have been. Your oncologist will explain the medicines and combinations you'll receive and their risks.

WHAT ABOUT IMMUNOTHERAPY, BONE MARROW TRANSPLANTS, AND EXPERIMENTAL TREATMENTS?

Oncologists sometimes recommend additional treatment for cancer patients. Here is some quick information about the various types.

Immunotherapy

Researchers have worked for decades to figure out how to trigger the body's immune system to fight or even prevent cancer. Two types of white blood cells fight infections: B lymphocytes and T lymphocytes. The B cells make the protein antibodies, or immunoglobins, that destroy foreign substances like viruses. The T cells recognize rogue cells and attack. Helper

Immunotherapy uses T cells to fight cancer. These special cells, called cytotoxic T cells, seek out and destroy defective or damaged cells without harming healthy ones.

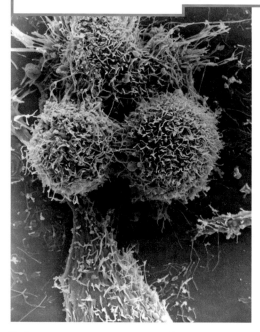

T cells regulate nearly all immune system activities. Three immunotherapy treatments have shown some promise.

Monoclonal antibodies are made by injecting human cancer cells or proteins from cancer cells into mice. Their immune systems create antibodies. The antibodies are removed and fused with laboratory-grown cells to create hybrid cells that can produce a lot of pure antibodies. Doctors inject the antibodies into cancer patients.

Injecting helper T cells is another form of immunotherapy. Helper T cells secrete cytokines. These cytokines can stimulate B cells to produce antibodies or enhance the cytoxic, or cancer-fighting, ability of certain T cells. Doctors use cytokines to enhance cancer patients' overall immunity. This form doesn't attack a specific cancer type.

Researchers have also developed tumor vaccines that activate T cells to seek out and attack certain proteins. The vaccines have shown some short-term successes with certain cancers. Like other cancer treatments, one form doesn't do the trick. Doctors use combinations of immunotherapy to fight cancer. And patients respond to immunotherapy as differently as they do chemo and radiation.

Bone Marrow Transplants

A bone marrow transplant (BMT) is an intensive form of immunotherapy. It's often the first thing doctors use to treat chronic myelogenous leukemia. It's also used for some lymphoma patients and leukemia patients who relapse, who don't respond to chemotherapy, or whose cancers are extremely high risk.

The first step is to find a donor. Ideally, if you need a BMT, you'll have a perfect match—someone with blood identical to yours. You'll have less chance of rejecting the marrow. Siblings are usually your best chance. They have a one in four shot at being a perfect match. Parents are usually half-matches. That's because you got half your genes from your mom and the other half from your dad. Genetics are tricky, though. You might even find a stranger is closer to your blood match than anyone in your family.

You can have a successful transplant without a perfect match, but the risks for complications are higher.

A simple blood test determines who will make a good match. Your doctor can give you information on testing possible donors. The bone marrow registry will also seek out the best possible match if you don't have a suitable sibling donor.

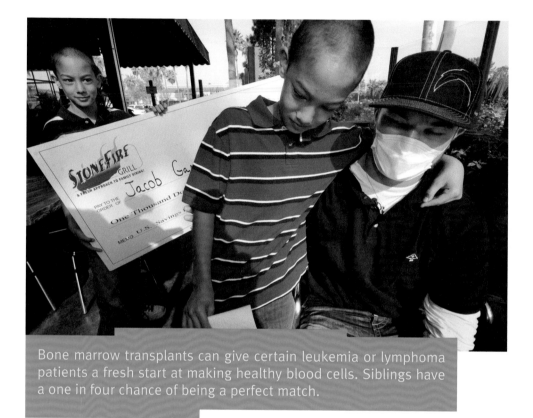

Bone marrow transplants can give certain leukemia or lymphoma patients a fresh start at making healthy blood cells. Siblings have a one in four chance of being a perfect match.

Once a transplant patient finds a donor, things move pretty quickly. First, doctors give preparative chemotherapy, which may also include total body irradiation. This treatment empties most of the bone marrow to make room for the new and healthy blood-forming stem cells from the donor bone marrow. Transplant patients usually need antibiotics and blood transfusions during this time.

Meanwhile, doctors prep the donor for harvest. Donors have presurgical blood tests and must fast before the harvest. Collecting bone marrow can actually be done one of two ways.

A real bone marrow harvest is done surgically to ensure complete sterility (lack of infection). Donors need general anesthesia during the procedure. In the operating room, doctors inject a special needle into the donor's hip to withdraw bone marrow. How much a doctor takes depends on how much the recipient weighs. For example, a 100-pound (45 kilogram) cancer patient will need about one hundred teaspoonfuls of bone marrow.

Taking out this much marrow won't harm the healthy donor. His or her body will replenish those cells pretty quickly. Donors report mild to moderate pain at the harvest site for a few days after the procedure. Painkillers and rest make them more comfortable.

Another type of bone marrow harvest does not involve taking actual bone marrow, but consists of collecting stem cells from the bloodstream. Donors who undergo a peripheral blood stem-cell harvest first take shots of a medicine to boost white blood cell production, which includes stem cells, for a few days. They'll then get special venous catheters placed to collect their stem cells. Donors are hooked up to a special machine for a few hours to filter their blood and remove mostly stem cells.

Stem cells for a transplant can also be obtained from umbilical cord blood. The umbilical cord is the long tube that connects a growing fetus to its food source, the placenta. When a baby is born, its umbilical cord can be saved and its blood "banked" in a freezer for future use. Umbilical cord blood is rich in stem cells.

Once the cancer patient is ready, doctors will inject healthy bone marrow, peripheral blood, or umbilical cord stem cells directly into the blood stream through the catheter. The goal is for the new cells to reproduce more healthy cells. The cells circulate, reproduce, and rebuild marrow after a period of growth. This is called engraftment. Patients usually need more blood transfusions in the next weeks or even months as their bodies rebuild the supply.

Some side effects of a BMT are similar to chemotherapy. Many patients feel sick to their stomachs. Medicine can help, but most people don't have much of an appetite for several days to weeks after their transplants. Food can taste different. Some people develop mouth sores. Because nutrition is so important during engraftment, doctors often opt to keep transplant patients on nutritional IVs or feeding tubes.

The first one hundred days after a BMT are the most important. The biggest risk is infection. It takes a good six to twelve months before the immune system is strong again. Transplant patients who develop fevers must be hospitalized and given antibiotics so that doctors can monitor for complications, like infections. Viruses and fungus infections can be dangerous, so patients usually take medicines after their transplants to prevent these infections.

Another big risk to bone marrow transplants is graft-versus-host disease (GVHD). This can occur within a few days of engraftment or even years later. GVHD that occurs shortly after the transplant is called acute GVHD. Patients can develop a skin rash, diarrhea, and liver problems. Chronic GVHD happens later. It can affect different body parts, including the skin, mouth, lips, and liver. GVHD is often treated with steroids, such as prednisone, to calm an overactive immune system.

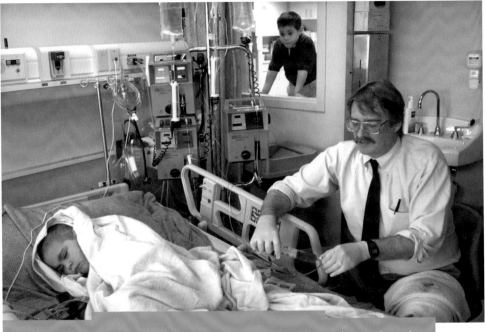

Bone marrow transplants are painless for cancer patients, but the preparation steps make them weak. It takes months for a body to rebuild its blood supply and immunity after a transplant.

Waiting for bone marrow to engraft takes a lot out of a body. Sometimes the body's organs do not work well while waiting. Blood pressure can rise because of poor kidney function. The liver might become swollen and tender. Poor liver function can cause jaundice, or a yellowing of the skin and eyes. Many of these conditions can be treated and will eventually end.

There's one last thing you need to know about BMT. The body must go through many aggressive steps to prepare for the procedure. Most people who have bone marrow transplants become sterile. They cannot have children. Talk to your doctor about the risks.

Experimental Treatments

Doctors don't offer experimental treatment options casually. In some cases, an oncologist might believe a cancer could respond to an experimental drug or procedure. In most cases, doctors have tried all possible available treatment options but a cancer won't respond.

Clinical trials are the last stage of approving experimental drugs or treatment methods for standard use. Researchers collect data from human patients to track the new treatment's effectiveness. There are successful outcomes, but experimental treatment does not always help every patient. Nonetheless, any patient who takes part in a clinical trial will provide crucial data that helps advance the future of cancer treatment.

Not all patients make good candidates. If your doctors recommend a trial, make sure they explain why they think this will be the best route. They should also fully explain the requirements. These can include cancers at a certain stage, previous treatments tried, an age range, and so on. Know the risks if you decide to try experimental treatments and the possible outcome if you refuse. The most important thing to remember: you can leave a clinical trial at any time. Your doctor can also choose to remove you if the treatment is not helping you or your side effects are too severe.

Ten Great Questions to Ask Your Doctor

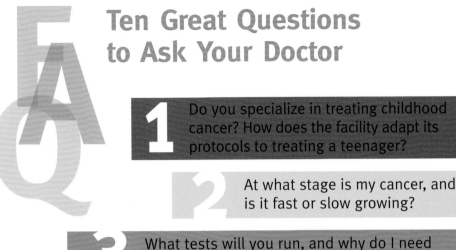

1 Do you specialize in treating childhood cancer? How does the facility adapt its protocols to treating a teenager?

2 At what stage is my cancer, and is it fast or slow growing?

3 What tests will you run, and why do I need them? What happens during those tests?

4 What are my treatment options, and how long will they last?

5 What are possible side effects? What medicines can I take to relieve side effects? Are there any risks to taking these medicines?

6 If I have surgery, how long will the operation and recovery last?

7 Will I need drains, catheters, other intra-venous lines, or blood transfusions?

8 Do I need to eat a special diet?

9 Will I still be able to do the activities and sports I love after treatment or surgery?

10 How soon must we decide on a treatment?

six

HOW WILL CANCER CHANGE LIFE AT HOME?

Cancer affects your entire family. Even the strongest ones struggle under its strain. Your parents and siblings might worry about how to talk to you about what you're going through. Parents may feel guilty that you got cancer—was it something they did or did not do? Very young children might worry that they caused their brother or sister to get cancer because they were mean or had a fight. Many parents of cancer patients admit they didn't want to talk about worst-case scenarios, late effects, and their fears. They figured their child had enough to deal with already.

And you do. The rest of your family has a lot to deal with, too. The more you know and understand what your family will go through, the better prepared your family will be to get through these next months together.

How Does My Cancer Affect My Parents?

If your parents could take your cancer into their own bodies, they would. The chaotic first weeks after a diagnosis are filled with restless nights for you and your parents. Like you, they spend their days trying to decipher complex medical terms. Like you, they feel overwhelmed by the decisions they face. Unlike you, they bear the burden of having the final say in your treatment until you turn eighteen. They have as many worries on their minds as you do right now, perhaps even more.

If you have younger siblings, your parents will be worried about how to explain your cancer to them in a way they can understand. Adults still must pay household bills, get other children to school, do laundry, and go to the grocery store. They worry about household viruses and bacteria that might harm you. They must balance the need to earn money to cover these new expenses with the need to be with you. If the nearest treatment center is far away, your parents must weigh the choices of disrupting the family and moving or splitting up the family while you and one of your parents move closer to the facility. They have to manage insurance, hospital, and medication paperwork. Single parents or those without family support have an even tougher time balancing the extra responsibilities.

Some parents of cancer patients admit they second-guessed themselves constantly and wished someone else could have told them what to do. Others say they became obsessed with learning all they could about treatment, thinking perhaps they could

A child's cancer diagnosis puts a huge strain on families. Honest communication, support from friends, and laughter will get you all through rough times.

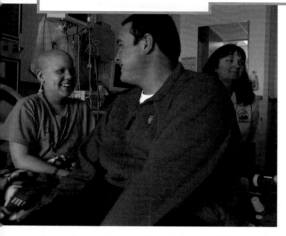

control the process. Some say they questioned God or lost their faith. Others clung to their religious teachings.

Your parents might react in different ways, but they will go through similar anguish. Many caregivers develop tunnel vision. They focus entirely on the illness and treatment and forget about themselves. Parents need to make time for each other, their other children, and their friends. Your social worker can talk to your family members about taking care of themselves as they care for you. They can lead you to helpful resources.

You can help, too. Encourage your parents to accept help from family and friends. Let them know they need to take time for themselves. If they protest, gently remind them that they are no help to you if they are completely stressed out.

Parent will also focus on your stomach, just as they did when you were a baby. Nutrition is extra important because your body is still maturing. You need food packed with vitamins, minerals, protein, and healthy fat to feed your cells so that they can recover from treatment and still grow.

The fact is you will likely have days when you don't want to eat. Your parents can become stressed on those days when you don't feel like eating. To you, it might seem like your parents are badgering you. Many families talk about how food became a huge stressor. Parents demanded, then begged, their children to eat. The children stubbornly stood their ground, frustrated and wishing their parents would leave them alone.

Talk to your parents and nutritional counselor now about the best way to handle appetite issues or potential problems that might pop up later. Together, you can develop a menu you'll want to eat and a plan to manage those days when food is the last thing you want. And you need to remember that nutrition is a top priority. It's your job to help your body be as healthy as it can. Protein, carbohydrates, and fat are your weapons.

How Does Cancer Affect Other Family Members and Friends?

In the coming months, the people who love you will feel like they are stuck on the sidelines. Siblings, grandparents, stepparents, other family members, and friends of cancer patients often feel helpless. They want to be part of the caregiving process but don't always know how.

Many people who've gone through the experience say they weren't sure at first how to act around the cancer patient. Would they say or do the wrong thing?

Brothers and sisters report feeling neglected at times by their parents or conflicted by their own feelings. Sometimes they resented the attention their sick sibling received. Sometimes they felt guilty because they were healthy. Sometimes they felt angry and wanted to yell, other times to hide and cry. Some children developed changes in their personality, such as becoming aggressive at school. Some withdrew from friends.

One decision you all must make is whether to see a family counselor. It might feel awkward at first, airing frustration or confusion to a stranger, but it can help. Family counselors can teach you how to best communicate strong emotions and fears.

If you have siblings, involve them in your care. When they know and understand what is happening to you, they will feel more confident in the future. This insight will create a strong sense of compassion and responsibility not just for you, but for all people. Most important, it will allow your siblings to cope during difficult times when your parents might be focused entirely on you.

Most people who've been through a family member's cancer say they felt most useful when they truly helped, however small. Accept help from those who offer it, and give them a task. Grandparents, aunts or uncles, and family friends can be a huge source of support. They can take care of daily chores or child care while your parents focus on you. They can be a mental break for you: there will be days when you want to talk about anything other than cancer, nutrition, blood counts, and treatments.

If you don't have strong family support, you can get help from your cancer team. Social workers, family counselors, and others can help you navigate through rough patches. They can put you in touch with community resources to help ease the burden.

Decades of research have led to more effective cancer treatments and medicines. Five-year survival rates for many childhood cancers average above 70 percent and are rising each year.

And What About Me?

Cancer does a number on your body, and it can do just as much damage mentally. Weight changes, hair loss, mouth sores, surgical scars, catheters—suddenly you have a whole new set of image issues. You'll

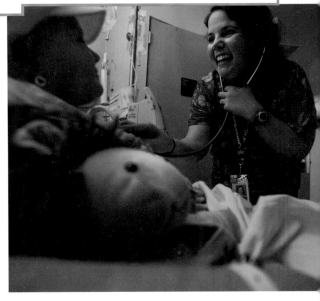

likely feel isolated because you must miss out on school activities, team events, or just playing around the neighborhood.

It's especially hard if you already feel self-conscious. Some families who've been through cancer recommend a schedule and limitations for visits. Decide now how you want to handle visits. It will make it easier on days when you feel worn down or stressed out.

Perhaps the most important decision you can make is how you are going to treat yourself. You now belong to a truly unique group. People want to help you, to welcome you and guide you. Trust yourself and others' good intentions. The support you get from your medical team, other cancer patients, and cancer survivors will be a lifeline during the toughest times ahead.

adjuvant therapy Therapy given after the primary cancer treatment to lower the likelihood that cancer will return.

alopecia Hair loss.

benign Something that is not harmful; noncancerous.

biopsy The removal of cells to examine them for diagnosis.

brachytherapy A form of radiation therapy in which radioactive isotopes are inserted in or on the surface of the body.

carcinogen Something shown to cause cancer.

carcinoma Cancer found in the tissues that line or cover organs.

catheter A tube inserted in the body to deliver medicines, allow blood draws, or facilitate drainage of fluid. A central venous catheter is placed surgically into a large vein and can be used to give chemotherapy.

hematologist A doctor who specializes in blood diseases.

idiopathic Something of unknown origin; can describe cancer cells or illnesses/complications that develop for unknown reasons.

immunotherapy Treatment designed to stimulate the immune system; also called biological therapy.

indolent Something that is slow-growing.

induction therapy The initial therapy used to treat cancer; often called first-line or primary treatment.

infiltrating or invasive cell A cancer cell that spreads to surrounding areas.

malignant Something that is harmful; cancerous.

metastasis The spread of cancer cells from the origin to other body parts.

oncologist A doctor who specializes in treating cancer.

palliative care Treatment to relieve cancer symptoms, such as pain, nausea, sores, etc.

prognosis An estimate regarding the outcome of cancer or other diseases.

protocol A treatment plan.

recurrence When cancer redevelops after remission.

remission The disappearance of cancer cells.

resection Surgical removal of a tumor.

sarcoma Cancer in the connective tissues, such as bone and cartilage.

American Cancer Society

P.O. Box 22538

Oklahoma City, OK 73123-1538

(800) ACS-2345 [227-2345]

Web site: http://www.cancer.org

The American Cancer Society is dedicated to eliminating and preventing cancer through research, education, and advocacy. The Web site offers links to insightful articles about treatment options, insurance and legal tips, and more.

Canadian Cancer Society

National Office

10 Alcorn Avenue, Suite 200

Toronto, ON M4V 3B1

Canada

(416) 961-7223

Web site: http://www.cancer.ca

The Canadian Cancer Society is a national community-based organization of volunteers. Its mission is the eradication of cancer and the enhancement of the quality of life of people living with cancer.

Children's Brain Tumor Foundation

274 Madison Avenue, Suite 1004

New York, NY 10016

(866) 228-HOPE [228-4673]

Web site: http://www.cbtf.org

The Children's Brain Tumor Foundation is a nonprofit organization founded in 1988 by dedicated parents, physicians,
and friends of cancer patients. It offers a monitored discus-
sion board, links to support groups, and more.

National Childhood Cancer Foundation

4600 East-West Highway, Suite 600

Bethesda, MD 20814-3457

(800) 458-6223

Web site: http://www.curesearch.org

The National Childhood Cancer Foundation can help patients
find a Children's Oncology Group institution in their area.
Information from some of the world's best pediatric cancer
specialists is available on its Web site.

Web Sites

Due to the changing nature of Internet links, Rosen Publishing
has developed an online list of Web sites related to the subject
of this book. This site is updated regularly. Please use this link
to access the list:

http://www.rosenlinks.com/faq/canc

For Further Reading

Blackman, Malorie, et al. *Shining On: A Collection of Stories in Aid of the Teen Cancer Trust*. London, England: Piccadilly Press, Ltd., 2006.

Block, Keith. *Life Over Cancer: The Block Center Program for Integrative Cancer Treatment*. New York, NY: Bantam, 2009.

Cutcher, Chris. *Deadline*. New York, NY: Greenwillow, 2007.

Dreyer, Zoann. *Living with Cancer* (Teen's Guides). New York, NY: Checkmark Books, 2008.

Grinyer, Anne. *Life After Cancer in Adolescence and Young Adulthood: The Experience of Survivorship*. New York, NY: Routledge, 2009.

Hilden, Joanne. *Shelter from the Storm: Caring for a Child with a Life-Threatening Condition*. Cambridge, MA: Da Capo Press, 2002.

Keene, Nancy, et al. *Childhood Cancer Survivors: A Practical Guide to Your Future*. Sebastopol, CA: O'Reilly Media, 2006.

Koss, Amy Goldman. *Side Effects*. New York, NY: Roaring Brook Press, 2006.

Schwartz, Cindy L., et al. *Survivors of Childhood and Adolescent Cancer: A Multidisciplinary Approach*. New York, NY: Springer, 2005.

Sullivan, Nanci A. *Walking with a Shadow: Surviving Childhood Leukemia*. Santa Barbara, CA: Praeger Publishers, 2004.

American Cancer Society. "Children Diagnosed with Cancer: Financial and Insurance Issues." Retrieved December 27, 2009 (http://www.cancer.org/docroot/CRI/CRI_2_6x_ financial_and_insurance_issues_7.asp).

American Cancer Society. "What Are the Types of Childhood Cancer?" May 19, 2009. Retrieved November 24, 2009 (http://www.cancer.org/docroot/ CRI/content/CRI_2_4_1X_What_are_the_types_of_ childhood_cancers_7.asp).

Cefrey, Holly. *Coping with Cancer*. New York, NY: The Rosen Publishing Group, 2000.

Kaufman, Howard, MD. "Immunotherapy for Cancer: A Continuing Medical Education Enduring Material." Medicine Online. Retrieved March 30, 2010 (http:// www.meds.com/immunotherapy/intro.html).

KidsHealth.org: Teen Health. "Types of Cancers Teens Get." June 2007. Retrieved November 24, 2009 (http:// kidshealth.org/teen/diseases_conditions/cancer/types_ of_cancer.html).

Leukemia & Lymphoma Society. "Childhood Blood Cancers." October 30, 2009. Retrieved November 24, 2009 (http://www.leukemia-lymphoma.org/all_page.adp? item_id=495199).

Leukemia & Lymphoma Society. "Facts and Statistics."
    July 1, 2009. Retrieved November 24, 2009 (http://www.
    leukemia-lymphoma.org/all_page?item_id=12486).
National Cancer Institute. "ACS: French Study Yields High
    Survival Rate for Children with Lymphoma, Leukemia."
    July 9, 2001. Retrieved December 15, 2009 (http://www.
    cancer.org/docroot/NWS/content/NWS_1_1x_French_Study_
    Yields_High_Survival_Rate_for_Children_With_Lymphoma_
    Leukemia.asp).
National Cancer Institute. "Bone Cancer: Questions and Answers."
    March 13, 2008. Retrieved December 13, 2009 (http://
    www.cancer.gov/cancertopics/factsheet/sites-types/bone).
National Cancer Institute. "General Information About
    Childhood Brain and Spinal Cord Tumors." October 15, 2009.
    Retrieved December 13, 2009 (http://www.cancer.gov/
    cancertopics/pdq/treatment/childbrain/Patient).
National Cancer Institute. "Radiation Risks and Pediatric
    Computed Tomography (CT): A Guide for Health Care
    Providers." December 22, 2008. Retrieved December 27,
    2009 (http://www.cancer.gov/cancerinfo/causes/radiation-
    risks-pediatric-CT).
National Cancer Institute. "Surveillance, Epidemiology, and
    End Results" (Tables on Childhood Cancer Incidence,
    Prevalence, Five-Year Survival, and Mortality Rates,
    Age-Adjusted from 1975–2006). Retrieved December 13,
    2009 (http://seer.cancer.gov).

Pui, Ching-Hon, et al. "Treatment of Childhood Acute Lymphoblastic Leukemia Without Cranial Irradiation," *New England Journal of Medicine*, Vol. 360, No. 26. June 25, 2009, pp. 2,730–2,741.

Steen, R. Grant, and Joseph Mirro, MD. *Childhood Cancer: A Handbook from St. Jude's Children's Research Hospital.* New York, NY: Perseus Publishing, 2000.

Stewart, Gail B. *The Other America: Teens with Cancer.* San Diego, CA: Lucent Books, 2002.

Woznick, Leigh A., and Carol D. Goodheart. *Living with Childhood Cancer: A Practical Guild to Help Families Cope.* Washington, DC: American Psychological Association, 2002.

Index

About the Author

Colleen Ryckert Cook is a writer for teens and an editor in Kansas City. Two of her classmates lost their fights with leukemia in 1978 and 1984. Today, the five-year survival rate for acute lymphocytic leukemia is nearing 90 percent. She hopes we can soon say the same about all cancers. Her father died from lung cancer in 2002. Her sister is a breast cancer survivor.

Photo Credits

Cover blue jean images/Getty Images; p. 6 MedicalRF.com/ Getty Images; p. 10 © Lezlie Sterling/Sacramento Bee/ZUMA Press; p. 13 © AP Images; p. 17 © Custom Medical Stock Photo; p. 20 © Simon Fraser/RVI, Newcastle upon Tyne/Photo Researchers, Inc.; p. 22 © www.istockphoto.com/Chris Hutchison; p. 25 © www.istockphoto.com/Mark Kostich; p. 27 © M.Bradford/CMSP; p. 34 © San Antonio Express-News/ ZUMA Press; p. 37 © Bob Larson/Contra Costa Times/ZUMA Press; p.40 Photolibrary/Getty Images; p. 42 © The Orange County Register/ZUMA Press; p. 45 krtphotos/Newscom.com; p. 50 © Kristopher Skinner/Contra Costa Times/ZUMA Press; p. 53 © Bryan Patrick/Sacramento Bee/ZUMA Press.

Designer: Evelyn Horovicz; Editor: Bethany Bryan; Photo Researcher: Amy Feinberg